# HAPPY HEAD

The "Spiritual" Guide to Amazing Oral
Sex

# JASMINE P. RAIN

Happy Head: The "Spiritual" Guide to Amazing Oral Sex

Definition of Euphoria (According to dictionary.com©)

1. A state of intense happiness and self-confidence.
2. A feeling of happiness, confidence, or well-being sometimes exaggerated in pathological states as mania.

Definition of Oral Sex (According to
dictionary.com©)


1. Sexual contact between the mouth
   and the genitals or anus:
   fellatio, cunnilingus, or
   anilingus




Dedication

I would like to thank my long-time friend of 15 years and my agent, Felicia, for continuing to believe in me. Even when my self-doubt began to kick into the speed of a 1970 Chevelle with a 450 horsepower engine... Words cannot express how grateful I am.

I also dedicate this book to all of my experiences, both "good" and seemingly "negative" because without them I would not have knowledge and wisdom.

Thank you to God, All-That-Is, my Angels and the ever-present holy energy that keep me grounded and happy with myself without judgment. I love myself and know that I've been placed in this world to live my Truth. My Truth... And no one else's...

Jasmine ♥

# Contents

Are You a Happy Head? Quiz

Author Info

# INTRODUCTION

Before you can begin to please another human being, you have to become comfortable with yourself first. Happiness should be essential to your life in a way that it takes precedence over everything. Without happiness and positive thinking, your life cannot manifest the things in life you desire. Money, career, peaceful living and relationships are all affected by your state of mind.

In relationships, much compromise is involved between two people in various ways. Sex can play a major role in whether or not the relationship can sustain at maximum level. It all depends on how important it is to each person. Frequency and the art of sex can be major players in the mind of one mate, but not so important to the other. My belief is to gain a full understanding of what your partner's needs are before committing to the relationship. That way, you can assess whether or not their desires, or un-desires, are something you can live with. This is very important because it can cause unwanted problems in the long haul. You guys may argue over petty things and not realize that those arguments are stemming from the sexual responses in the relationship. This can create a subconscious resentment that could damage the union.

Once you begin to realize the love of yourself and how it connects to the love of your relationship, pleasure will come naturally.

When it comes to sex, I happen to favor fellatio, or more commonly known as oral sex or "giving head". I am not quite sure of the reasoning behind the enjoyment it has for me, but I know it has much to do with my love of penis. When I was younger, my mother told me that sex was not "good" and that it was a waste of time. She either was trying to protect me from getting pregnant at an early age or she really had some distaste for sex. It had to quench her thirst at some point in life being that my sister and I are here. However, when I was thirteen, I recall lying in my bed half asleep and hearing my mother and her boyfriend knocking the headboard against the wall of our 2 bedroom apartment. I knew from the many movies I'd seen, that I'm most certain I wasn't supposed to be watching, that the female made moaning sounds while engaging in sex. It seemed to be a natural part of the process. While listening to wood bang against sheetrock, not a sound seeped from the vocal chords of my mother. Not one sound... It was broad daylight, so maybe she was thinking about us kids...

In that same apartment one late night while my sister and I were sleeping, the same scenario but now with my mother and her "best girlfriend", Daisy, I could hear the squealing sounds of passionate wails wafting through our four walls. I screamed to the top of my hormonal lungs and then my mother came storming through me and my sister's door without clothes. "Are you gay?!" Those were the first words that I could muster although I already knew the answer to my own question. That night forever changed my life and my view of sexuality. Unlike my mother, I love sex and I'm 99.9% certain that it will be top priority in my life well into my old age.

For me, there's nothing like the sight of an erect nature made muscle, loaded with veins, flowing with the blood that sustains the very essence of physical human life. There is power in a penis. Amazingly, it has a head, one good eye and two "legs" to hold it up when it gets excited. I would much prefer a penis over a kitty cat any day, but that is my preference. And toys won't cut it for me. Nothing fake, glass or plastic, can be high powered enough to stimulate this pussy cat. I need the real deal in that the connection is not just with the shaft but also with the person the shaft belongs to...

I wrote this book because of my love of the art of oral stimulation. My love for it has always been natural and I've found that when I truly love something, it's not a chore. It's something that I could be "working" on, without any realization of the time lapse. You know when you've been doing something and all of a sudden you realize that hours have passed? You weren't focused on the time because you were enjoying whatever you were doing. Passion is the best word to describe this feeling.

Although oral sex is something that happens behind closed doors, I am in no way ashamed to express my love for it, as it is an extension of the giving aspect of my innate personality.

Sex for me is one of the ultimate aphrodisiacs. I can lose myself in its moments and catch myself with an ethereal smile on my face. It's euphoria at its best. Then my brain speaks, "I see lions, mountains and trees... Rainbows... Maybe even fairy stardust..." It is common for me during many of my excursions to yell out in the loudest voice I can muster, "Omg, this is euphoria!" So if having intercourse has that effect on me, then I have to explain how sucking my guy's penis throws me into a state of a euphoric unconsciousness...

From my first sexual encounter, I found myself with my face lying on the inside of my guy's thigh, staring at his erect penis. I wanted to become one with it and from that first oral contact, I knew exactly the "right" way to please him. The energy exuded from the spiritual connection between him and I enabled me to go into a deep space, without any need for pleasure in return. As a matter of fact, I am a terrible receiver...

I am not too fond of receiving "head," as it feels weird to me. Something about a wet tongue in my vulva doesn' t get me aroused. I' m not going to say that I have never enjoyed it, but I can definitely take a rain check. Maybe it has something to do with my mother being a lesbian. But even if that was not the case, I still don' t think I would enjoy the slosh feeling of saliva marinating down there...

In terms of the "deep space" I made reference to earlier, I' ve always referred to myself as "blanking out" during the act because I don' t focus on any thoughts but the task at hand. It' s like driving and forgetting to get off at your exit because you' re in a zone. "Do you remember what you did when you were sucking my dick? I want you to do it again..." is what my guy would ask.

"No" is always my response because I'm constantly in a deep connection with the very important energy exchange involved with my passion.

When I'm sucking my guy's penis in the car is when my consciousness tends to fade more so than ever. It's such a thrill to hold onto your guy's penis with one hand with your mouth attached while his foot is trying to follow only one side of his brain. The power is invigorating!

For decades, a tabooed stigma has been attached to oral stimulation. While rarely enforced, it has been considered a felony in the law books of some states in the U.S. As a teenager growing up in the hormonal sexual years, most girls my age were saying that oral sex was off limits for them. If penis entered your mouth, you were viewed as being "nasty". Although I was not that sexually active, the one boyfriend I did have definitely knew my fetish. Even at that age, I didn't give two flying saucers what others thought. That passion I had for "giving head" carried into my adult years, thus the reason for this manual.

This book is not only birthed out of my own personal passion, but also out of conversations with several women who have expressed to me that they do not have any desire to please their guy orally. However, they've expressed that it is necessary to keep their relationship alive. Borderline mandatory... Some women feel that oral sex is disgusting or less than pleasing to them. It makes them want to gag even thinking about putting a penis in their mouth. Then there are those women who have a desire to please their guy, but feel as though when they attempt the act, they are not performing it correctly. The common denominator: Both groups want someone to show them how to "give head" passionately and how to do it well. This manual is a step by step guide to pleasing your guy with enough passion to satisfy you both.

# Chapter 1

## Connecting With Yourself

Every day we all wake up and walk around in our given or "chosen" bodies. At an early age, we develop a desire to wash, clothe and feed ourselves so that we may innately connect with "Us". Our brains produce thoughts that we may only know, unless of course, we choose to share with others. Ultimately, we live a life nurturing our bodies through the five senses: Sight, Taste, Touch, Audibility and Smell. At the top of the "sense" list is touch. Whether or not we can see or develop a temporary loss of the ability to taste or hear, we all have the deep desire to be touched. It is a natural occurrence in all species on this planet we call Earth.

From basic gardening to the art of horticulture, research shows that plants have a greater ability to thrive in a place where other plants are near. Even just talking to a plant or giving it extra attention can make it grow to be a wildebeest. When I lived in Florida, I started planting Marigolds just to see if I could keep a flower alive. When I succeeded with those, I added another flower and then another, until finally I had a huge garden! I would spend hours tending to the garden and the more attention I gave it, the bigger the plants grew.

When I dug my hands in the soil, I could feel the connection I had to the earth. That initial trusting of my inner self to connect with something new grew into a lifelong passion. People would come by my home just to view the garden that I created. That connection allowed others to connect in their own way.

The same goes for animals, especially caged birds. A bird all alone in a cage without touch from a human or another bird can make it depressed. My experience with my lonesome dove was enough to drive me crazy. I saw the sadness in his eyes. I could no longer watch it all alone in a cage. I knew that I could not manage two birds, not with all the feces it likes to create. I contemplated letting it fly free in the wind, but then I knew that it may not survive long. So I gave it away to a more attentive home. My family thought I was crazy for thinking the dove had feelings, but I could feel its pain. I could feel the connection...

Plants, animals and humans all crave a connection with something or someone. No one wants to be alone, no matter what they say. People die from loneliness because there's a dis-connect somewhere in their lives. We can all benefit from learning to become better at connecting with everything we do. It's essential.

When there is a lack of the ability to be touched by another person, we have the tools to satisfy the need on our own. We know our bodies better than anyone else. We breathe, eat and sleep in them. We bathe and oil ourselves with the hands attached to our own bodies. Although we desire to connect with others, we are very capable of being self-sufficient. Sometimes we need to dis-connect from the outside world, even if just for minutes, so that we can re-connect with ourselves. It's like recharging a battery so

that it can aggressively fuel the thing it
needs to power. Taking a nice, hot shower or
long bubble bath, allowing yourself to
daydream, reading, staring at the clouds or
maybe getting a mani/pedi can relax you
enough to remember who you are as your own
person. There's the saying that "You can't
help anyone else until you help
yourself..." Put the oxygen mask on your face
first. I guarantee your connection to the
outer world will be much brighter...

Meditation and yoga are great tools in
helping to get in touch with our inner selves
whether it is spiritually, intellectually or
sexually. That attunement to "All-That-Is"
will help you to better connect with another
with effortless behavior. Not only will you
connect with others but with everything
around you. Your senses will become much
clearer and you will have a more open view of
your surroundings. There are many ways to
meditate or connect. Prayer, silent
meditation, or just being alone in your
thoughts can be great ways to come unto
yourself. It opens the airwaves to the
universe. Eating healthy and exercising

regularly can also make you feel better about yourself emotionally and physically. This will no doubt have a more positive affect on your outer relationships.

Self-stimulation in matters of sex is pertinent in order to get better acquainted with your body as well. What better way to get to know the response of the human body than to do research on yourself? Masturbation can help with knowing which sensations are pleasing to the cells so when someone else touches you, you already know what you do or don' t like. It pains me to hear people say that they don' t like to touch themselves sexually or that masturbation is a sin. At the age of fourteen, I began masturbating. My mother would leave porn videos on top of the TV, so naturally my curiosity gave way to watching them. I learned how to masturbate by watching women do it on the videos, not to mention, my hormones were raging. It felt so good and even at that age, seemed to be a release of tension from every day worries.

Take a few moments to touch yourself in your most private spot. Feel the sensations sway happily as if they were blades of grass flowing with the wind. These feelings are natural. If you can' t touch yourself, how do you expect to have someone else comfortably touch you?

Also, take a look in the mirror at yourself. You are beautiful. Whatever you think about yourself is going to be exuded from you when you come into contact with others. Being comfortable with the very essence of "who you are" is an important aspect of being comfortable with another human being. There has to be a connection first with yourself before you can intimately connect with another.

Chapter 2

Connecting With Your Mate

Energy is all around us. Every day we come into contact with our co-workers, the grocer, and that life-saving server at Starbucks. We sit on the roads in our cars to and from work and become one with traffic. We see the same faces during our daily commute on the train and telepathically try to pick their brains, wondering who they are outside of our perceptions of them. And then there are our neighbors... Although they may be separated from us by driveways or paper thin walls and may not necessarily be a direct part of our personal lives, we say our "hellos" and "goodbyes" and we know in some way we connect with them.

A lot of effort goes into making our day go smoother on a subconscious level. So why not develop a closer connection to your mate?

I'm a firm believer that even in the roughest of relationships; miracles can happen that can turn the relationship back into the exciting adventure it was when you guys first met. It happens to all of us. The beginning of a relationship can be a bushel of roses but can then wither as time passes. You both have to add fireworks to the pot to allow the bush to grow to its full potential. It takes two willing and loving spirits, meditation, prayer and some spark flying sex in order to make it work. Keeping that connection to yourself from the first chapter will make it easier to connect on a deeper level to your mate. As long as you have at least a college level understanding of yourself, you can at least gain an elementary understanding of the love of your life.

Take time during the day to call with your sexiest voice to just say hello or send a text saying "I love you". Or send him a sexy picture to get him aroused for what may happen when you meet later that evening. Leave all the troubles of the day at the door, preferably the back door, because bringing them into your relationship will only create unnecessary tension. He has already had to deal with troubles in his day, so adding two negatives will only make one enormous negative.

Let your guy know how handsome he is and how you appreciate his presence. Guys love to be appreciated, especially when they are putting forth the effort to sustain an honest relationship. Make him a surprise special dinner with candles. Or if you are a bit challenged in that area, order a meal from his favorite restaurant. Either way, he will know that you put in a great effort to please him. Rub your guy's back after a long day of work and ask him how his day went. With listening ears and little interruption, let him know how important he is to you by staring into eyes. There is nothing like deeply staring into the eyes of someone that you truly love. Hold hands when you guys are out in public. It's foreplay more than you will ever imagine. Not only will the two of you feel your connection, others will clearly see it and lust with envy.

It can be quite exciting to take a cruise or a day trip to get away from the mundane stressors in life. Family, kids, work, friends... They can all play a part in creating stress, but that can always be renewed. Plan to explore the world together. There is so much to discover outside of your everyday lives. You can never be too busy to add some excitement to your life, especially in a relationship.

No matter how conservative your guy may be, he will crave the excitement of a "newfound" partner. Just as you discover something new about yourself every day, by being more attentive to your partner you can find a different treasure hidden beneath the cruise ship of your love. You don't want it to set sail into the sea to never return... So keep the fireworks aflame in your relationship as much as you can or maybe even skydive from that plane thousands of feet up in the air. The adrenaline rush will keep you both alive. Who cares what people think? I say every time you live a life, LIVE IT to the fullest!

## Chapter 3

## Sensual Kisses

Kisses are a form of affection between two individuals that care about one another. There are different forms of kisses that demonstrate the type of relationship. Every day we see friends kissing friends, mothers pecking away at their children and partners drooling on each other. We even see the exchange between humans and their beloved animals. However, in some cultures kissing is taboo. On the flip side, in other cultures, it is common for it to be the preferred greeting for everyone. Either way, whatever the form, kissing has a loving stigma attached to it. I can guarantee that you will not be putting your lips on someone that you don't have some type of love for.

I've always loved the idea of kissing. I remember when I was around the age of 12, watching a movie and seeing a couple kiss and hoping one day that would be me. I could feel the energy of the kiss, even though it was

through a work of fiction. I knew at that age
that I wanted to have that passion in my
life. So when I became older, I kissed my
boyfriends with extreme reverence. It was
energetic, it was fun and I knew at some
point if I didn't stop, it would lead to
something else. The older I became, the more
it did.

My ex-husband never liked to kiss. I knew
this fact when we began dating, but allowed
his other qualities to outweigh it. When I
would go to kiss him, he would either turn
his head or peck me on the lips. It was
frustrating, to say the least, but I was
willing to take a loss for the team. At
first, I thought he had an issue with me, but
then he expressed his dislike for kissing.
More so, the exchange of tongues... It was a
great compromise for me, all the way to the
end of our marriage, twelve years later. I
was inexperienced. When I began dating other
people, I felt like a kissing newbie... What
had I been missing all those years? Maybe
that's one reason our marriage ended in
divorce. Either way, I enjoyed the re-

ignition of passion through kissing again and the endless possibilities seemed delicious.

Kissing is a form of connection with your partner. It can send the neurotransmitters in the brain into erotic robots. There is something about a soft and sensual kiss that can stir the blood in a way that it swirls around as if it were a patch of leaves on a wild and windy autumn day.

As Humans, we have a fascination with things that are soft. We want our fluffy pillows; our sheets a high thread count, the toilet tissue like clouds and our skin as smooth as porcelain. I don't blame us... It just feels good. So the same goes for kissing. It should be done in stages. I believe that if you begin a kiss sensually, you allow the energy to build for grand anticipation.

Make a point to kiss your partner whenever you greet each other. Hug him and run your fingertips along his back. Be sure that there is always a connecting intent. There is nothing like the feeling of being loved. Whenever you are "in the moment" with each other, it makes it easier for the sexual passion to be more intense.

Begin by looking into the eyes of your partner and placing your lips on his with loving intent. Make sure your lips are succulently moisturized. Your guy may love you but will definitely not want to kiss hard, chapped lips. Keep it sexy. Slowly kiss him with full lips on the mouth and then nibble at his bottom lip. Make your way to the side of his mandible (the edge of his jaw) and slowly kiss all the way to his neck and ears. Keep it soft and sensual and add some tongue. Grab his head and face with your hand and fingers while kissing him passionately. The level of energy should reach a high plane to the point that you can feel the heat and a tingling sensation in your body. At this point, you should begin to feel his "hardness" nudging you. Grab it and rub him there as you increase the level of the kiss. If you are a wild child, you may be a little more aggressive as you guys feverishly suck each other's faces off. It all depends on your personalities. The ultimate goal is to build up the energetic level of arousal to enter the next stage of passion.

Chapter 4

## Learning To Use the Muscles of Your Mouth (+Lips)

Using our mouths is a major part of our daily lives. We chew our food, brush our teeth, talk and breathe through it and depending on our different personalities, I'm sure there are a myriad of other uses not mentioned here. So without the muscles in our mouth, I'm thinking that it would be much harder for us to sustain life.

Our mouth muscles are naturally strong and capable of being malleable to whatever enters it. If you were to place an entire orange in your mouth, although it may be quite uncomfortable, the muscles in the mouth will be able to withstand it. The same goes for a penis. Depending on the size or shape of your mouth and/or the size and shape of your guy's penis, you can train your muscles to grasp it for full stimulation.

Much like Kegel exercises for the vagina, you
want to exercise your mouth muscles on a
regular basis. I suggest one of two things
(or both) in preparing for your guy. Take a
plantain, which is firmer than a banana, and
gently place it in your mouth. Close your
eyes and think of your guy (or any guy you
have a great affection for) and massage the
muscles in your mouth with the fruit. Let
your mouth gradually grip the plantain
tighter as your lips form together to make
the letter "O" . The masseter or jaw muscles
of your mouth should sink inwards as you
slide the plantain in and out of your mouth.
Move the plantain around the different zones
of your mouth. Take a moment to hold the
fruit in your mouth and count to ten as your
mouth firmly holds it in place. As you slowly
slide the plantain out of your mouth, pull
your lips together to make a smaller "O" as
the plantain leaves your mouth.

Your lips play a major role in creating a
massive sensation around the penis,
particularly the head. Repeat these exercises
until you are comfortable gripping the
plantain tightly with ease. It is important

that you practice these exercises without using your teeth. You want to treat the penis as if you were a lady having a dinner meeting. You wouldn't let your teeth scrape up against a utensil in a business meeting, would you? So don't let it happen with your guy's penis. Can you imagine being nipped in a sensitive area of your body with a sharp tooth? You know that feeling when you bite your own tongue? Not pretty... Unless of course your guy expresses to you that he likes for you to take a nibble here and there...

If you are not keen on using a piece of fruit to practice with and your guy is willing to allow you to practice on him, then why not? He may enjoy watching you progress from an eager amateur into that all-star professional. They say, "Practice makes Perfect," right?

Chapter 5

Tongue Lord

Our tongue is a very important asset to our mouth. Without it, it would be quite difficult to do the simplest things. The tongue is a strong muscle which holds a mass of cells that help us to have a sense of taste. Just as the tongue is a great asset for the enjoyment of food, it is your best friend when it comes to sucking the penis of your guy.

Using your favorite dildo for this exercise, preferably a flexible, non-glass one, start at the base with the tip of your tongue. Try to keep your tongue as moist as possible. As you work your way up the side of the apparatus, now with the flat part of your tongue, play around the shaft and feel for the veins. Pretend that they are the real veins on the penis of your guy. Remember: the veins connect to the heart and the bigger they get, the more the blood is flowing because of arousal. Once you' ve played

around on the playground for a while, you
want to use your tongue to lick around the
corona or ridge of the "King". That's
right, I said it... The KING... The head of
the penis is the top dog because it is where
all sensation for you and your guy lies. I
personally like a head that is quite
prominent in nature, which means it is very
well defined. I've been told that I have a
fascination with heads and not just the
penile type either. If you were to come to my
house, you would see that I have all kinds of
head sculptures placed around everywhere. So
yes... I literally have a head fetish.

Now back to the tongue... Put some love in
your lick. The more love and passion that you
put into what you're doing will be exuded in
your actions. Continue to lick around the
edges of the head and make your way to the
top. Lick it as you would lick any other part
of your man's body. Use your lips to make an
"O" and place them on the entire head while
using your tongue to swirl around. This is
where the work of multi-tasking begins. Let
your tongue be free to play around but have
some purpose. There is a urethral slit on the

head of the penis that you can opt to take a dive in, but it is your preference. You can stick your tongue deep inside or just lick around the surface of the hole. This is a very sensitive area, so you want to be gentle. Continue to make your way up and down the shaft with your tongue with vivacious spirit. Don't forget to show the testes or "balls" some tongue love, but we will explain that in detail in a later chapter.

The most important thing you can do when sucking on your guy's penis is to allow your tongue to be alive in combination with your lips and the muscles of your mouth. Be creative with your tongue. You can use the tip, the center, the sides, or if you have a massive tongue, why not use the whole thing? The key is to have lots of fun with it. The tongue is the "Lord" of the mouth when it comes to the art of sucking, so use it to your advantage.

Chapter 6

"Head" of the Household

"Head" is dirty work. There is no real way to "give head" with class. At least not in the traditional sense in which society views the definition... We are Humans but we are also animals by nature. Yes, there are some animals that are considered to be docile but then there are those others that are considered beasts. It's not that they are beasts 24 hours a day/7 days a week... They control when they feel like acting out aggressively. I believe we all have that control.

Some people may view "giving head" as a form of being submissive to your man. That could very well be true, but for me it is pure enjoyment. I have to be honest when I say that I do like being submissive at times, but I also like the sense of control that it can create. It all depends on your level of thinking. What truly matters is that you and your partner are connected and are allowing the pleasure to be received without hesitation.

There's so much power in the head of a penis. During sex, it is the first thing in and the last thing out. So it always gets the first and last feeling in the art of penetration. Semen or "cum" exits through the head and gives it a powerful, explosive sensation. The head equates to a clitoris on a woman. When the clitoris is aroused, it becomes somewhat hard and when the vagina "cums" to its satisfaction, the clitoris becomes sensitive. The head on a penis acts in the same way, so you want to treat it with care.

As I explained in an earlier chapter, the head is the King of the penis. The larger it gets in size, the more excited it has become. During the act of sex, this can be a great benefit for you both. This is why I like to "give head" first before indulging in the pleasure of sex.

After the sensual kisses in Chapter 3, slowly kiss your way down your guy's chest until you reach his pants. Begin to unbuckle his belt and unzip his pants. Let them drop to the floor and remove his boxers (if he wears them). The ideal picture that you want painted in your face is a nice, solid hard penis. If that is the case, watch it stare you in the face. In a few moments, it's going to become your best friend.

Let your mouth get wet with anxious anticipation as you grasp the head with your "O" shaped mouth. Grab the penis with your strongest hand and hold it with purpose. Let your tongue slide around the head as your lips pucker like the lips of a fish. Lick around the sides of the penis but don't take the whole thing in your mouth just yet. You want to be a little bit of a tease as you build up anticipation as well as the unknown on his end. After you have licked the sides, revert back to the head and with your mouth intently formed, continue to suck on it as if you are sucking the head of a lollipop. Lick around the edges of the head and in the urethral hole. This part is quite sensitive and could send your guy into frenzy, so be

prepared! You want to always be in control.
This is your domain...

## Chapter 7

## For the Guy Who Likes It Soft

Every guy is different. What may work for one may not cut it for the next. We all have our unique preferences when it comes to things and sex is no exception. There are fetishes that guys have that would probably blow your mind, but they learn to suppress them. They know most women would not be able to fully understand the "dirtiness" of their brains, so they may live out their fantasies secretly through porn.

There is nothing wrong with porn, in my opinion, just as long as there are no minors involved. Have you ever watched two people show affection by kissing and hugging in public? If so, you were watching an action of love. And if you are an advocate of love, it is a beautiful thing. I feel the same way about porn. If you love sex, what's so inappropriate with watching others doing the same thing that you love to do? Ideas are being exchanged to help spice up your life.

Go to the sexual fantasy store with your guy and peruse the aisles together to discover new toys. Pick out DVD's that you both will enjoy and don't be afraid to be open-minded. This field trip will not only get your creative juices flowing, but will also help you to better connect with your mate.

Watch porn when you are alone to help you to become comfortable, if you are not already, with the idea of it. It will help you to gain more of an understanding of yourself sexually. You will already have played out in your mind what you are willing and not willing to do before you engage in watching with your guy.

By watching porn, I discovered things about myself that I would've never known if I had not been open to watching. I now know that I have a fetish for watching threesome videos, but only with two guys and a girl. I also know that shockingly enough, I enjoy watching three guys, but only if one guy is sucking another. Well... I have to clear my throat on that one but I have to be honest. It's not that I really want to experience these movie fetishes, but that they stimulate me further for greater excitement in my own porn movie. There are no judgments, only pure and absolute mental fun.

Porn is like a visual manual. Sort of like this book... So I suggest watching porn with your guy, if he likes it. Watch it while sucking him. He will be turned on beyond excitement knowing that you are as freaky as he. However, you first have to be confident in yourself or else you will take one look at some of those women, and lose all self-esteem. You are not them and they are not you. It's pure entertainment.

Know your guy. When you are sucking, most guys will tell you their preference. Some are more vocal than others. From my personal experience, guys that like their penis to be rubbed gently will be more likely to want a "soft suck" . So you want to be a little gentler than what you may see on a porn video.

When sucking on this guy's penis, allow your mouth to be loose. Form that "O" but with not much effort. Inhale and exhale air with your lips pursed on his penis. With this guy, you want to lick and suck on his head with care. Follow the instructions for sucking the head in Chapter 6, but relax your mouth. Let the head gently hit the ridge of your upper palate. Activate your tongue and lips around the head with a mild suck.

Lick the sides of the penis with long and light strokes with just a little bit of pressure. Swallow the shaft whole with loose jaw muscles and gentle lips. Suck it as if you are sucking your thumb. Go up and down his shaft with twisting and turning motions, making sure to hit the ridge of your palate. Hold the base of his penis while you suck, up and down, coming up with sensual lips on the head. Begin to gradually massage the base of his penis while you suck but for this guy, you want to keep it light. This combination will make him harder, which is a result you want.

If your guy is not hard when you begin to suck his penis, take some cocoa butter or any natural oil/cream and rub him until he becomes engorged. Put your mouth on his head and just focus on that for a while. Continue to massage the shaft as you suck. Take your other hand and massage the area just under his head (about 2-3 inches down) in a twisting motion. Suck and twist gently, up and down with your thumb and index finger. Penetration of that area in combination with a good suck of the head will make your guy hard for sure. Continue practicing this knock out combo and you will be a "pro" in no time.

## Chapter 8

## For the Guy Who Likes It Hard

Some guys like it rough. Some girls do, too but that's another book. Guys are full of testosterone and need to play on the football field in everything they do. It's their way of letting off steam from all the stressors of life. They need to be reminded that they are indeed men, and so being a little aggressive during sex can really keep a guy calm. I don't care how conservative your guy, at some point he is going to want to have some rough sex. Don't take it personal.

When I was in school for Massage Therapy, most people did not want the traditional, relaxing "Swedish" massage. They wanted you to dig in the depths of their aching muscles to somehow numb the pain. As a massage therapist-in-training, your own muscles need to be strong enough to accommodate the request. Your hands and back need to be strong, so you have to make sure you are in tip top shape in order to provide for others.

With any type of "service", one has to be prepared for the job.

If your guy likes for his penis to be rubbed hard, then that is more indication that he will like to be sucked in the same manner. You want to get your jaws ready for this one. Ok... Let's stretch!

With this guy, you can begin a mild suck and then work your way to intensity. Think of it like a vigorous workout. You don't start off beating up your body immediately, but yet it is a gradual process. Whether you are on the bed or on the floor, get on your knees. This position will allow you to feel more in control. If you're on the floor, get a pillow or something padded so your knees won't feel uncomfortable. You could be there for a while.

Hold your guy's penis with both hands with the purpose I spoke about earlier. Place one hand at the base and the other in the middle of the shaft. Prepare your mouth with loads of saliva, which we will talk about in more detail in a later chapter. Suck the head with a tightly shaped "O" and a strong tongue. Massage his shaft with both hands as you suck on the "King". Use a twisting motion, as if you are wringing out a towel. You may elect to use your whole hand or just your index finger and thumb. The feeling your guy will receive is contingent upon the pressure of your stroke while still sucking.

With your hand strokes still in place, open your mouth wide enough to take a dive on your guy's whole penis and come back up. Keep sucking him whole, but make sure to come up to the head with each suck. Your jaws should be tightly squeezed inward, grasping the penis as if they have been best friends for years. You may feel your cheeks burning, but with practice this will dissipate. Your connection with yourself and your mate will greatly come into play at this time. You don't want to focus on the "work". The focus should be on enjoying yourself "in the moment" and pleasing your guy.

Grab the penis with your tongue and tight lips with the head hitting the top of your gums, up and down with saliva coating the penis. Continuous light to deep pressure, twisting with your mouth as if you are sucking on a lollipop... Make love to it. Don't give the appearance that you are suffering because he will notice. This will make his penis go a little soft, unless he is a guy that likes a girl in bondage. But for the most part, look your guy in the eyes with enjoyment.

Grab the base of his penis and suck on his shaft hard and slow while massaging the base. Come up to the head and suck as hard as you can and twist the part of the penis just under the head (2-3 inches) with vigor. Lose yourself in the moment. Don't focus on the time. It will reflect in your work. Don't think about throwing up either. Guys like the "throw up" or gag reflex sound. But even if that is a main concern for you, there are numbing aids for that issue. They come in different flavors and you can pick them up at any sexual fantasy store or online.

If you are like me and are not into using "helping agents", learn how to control the muscles in your throat. It takes practice.

You can practice regularly by sticking your
index finger in the back of your throat, just
enough but not so far back that you actually
throw up. You are training the muscles in
your throat to get accustomed to something
being in that place. If you are uncomfortable
with this exercise, then take advantage of
some practice while brushing your tongue with
your toothbrush. Go a little further back on
the tongue than usual. You will gag but this
will help with the training process.

Now take a trip to the testicle or "ball"
area. We talk about them in the next chapter.
Blow on them and let them know that they have
not been forgotten. There is a strip just
below the balls and right above the anus
called the perineum. For a lot of guys, this
area is an aphrodisiac. While sucking, you
can place a finger there and apply a bit of
pressure. Your guy may or may not like it
since it is quite close to the anus and some
guys are sensitive about that area. They may
even allow you to stick a finger in the anus
while you suck. You won't know until you
try...

Multitasking is going to always be the key in the process of "giving head". "Good head" ... The ultimate goal is to make your guy explode.

## Chapter 9

## Let's Play Ball

The "balls" are a sensitive area for guys. They house all the fruits of our creative world, which make them an important asset to human life. In the media you hear all types of jokes about it. The first thing a woman says when she is planning on hurting a guy is "I'm going to kick him the balls" ! We all know the preciousness of this area. Enter with caution.

Rub the balls of your guy with loving intention. They may feel rough or they may feel smooth. They may even have a fairly massive amount of hair on them. It depends on your guy. I like to sit and just watch my guy's ball as the sperm moves around in them. It's an amazing sight to me!

You may choose to grab the balls in your hands while you are sucking. Your guy may like them to be grabbed gently or he may like them manhandled. I've even known guys who

like to have them kicked. Every guy is
different. But just as a basic exercise, hold
them in the palm of your hand and swirl them
around using your thumb and fingertips as if
you are gripping a massage ball.

During oral sex, you may want to begin
sucking the balls first or go straight for
the penis. I usually go straight for the
penis, but it depends on the day. If I want
to send my guy over the edge with crazy
anticipation, I start with the balls as a
level of foreplay. It's like a warm-up
before the actual competition.

If you choose to begin with them first, take
the tip of your tongue and begin to lick
around the balls. Lick gently. You are
introducing yourself to them. Then casually
incorporate your lips as if you are French
kissing them. Kiss all around the bases and
then grab and massage on your guy's penis as
you lick his balls. Let your mouth get sloppy
wet with saliva as you juggle them in your
mouth, making sure your tongue is active.
Elect to swallow them whole in your mouth and
suck on them like you are sucking the head of

his penis. Place your hand just under them to hold them up while you suck. Juggle them with one hand; massage the shaft with another with your mouth on top. You are a pro at its finest with all those moves!

Bend your head deeper just under the balls and lick the perineum area. Start at the beginning of it, right near the anus, and bring your tongue up the middle of the balls towards the top of them in one long stroke. Continue with that stroke, if your guy desires it. Suck the balls again, go up and show the penis some love and apply pressure to the perineum at the same time. Some guys will love this!

You can play around with the balls in this same manner in the middle of your penis sucking session. It's all up to you in how you choose to incorporate the lessons. This is your play area. You are the boss.

Chapter 10

Saliva at Its Finest

Our mouths house a special liquid that help to break down the food that enters it. It is secreted from the pores of our mouths every second. That special liquid is called saliva or more commonly known as spit.

Its free lubrication has a variety of uses. It can lick the blood off a wound, wipe the crud from an eye or temporarily moisturize ash from your skin. During the act of oral stimulation, spit can become another one of your best friends. Sucking a penis with no lubrication would be quite odd, not only for the penis but for your mouth as well.

A few years ago, I went to the dentist and asked them if they could absorb some of the saliva from my mouth. I had never before had a problem with an overload of spit in my mouth, but for some reason secretions were in abundance. The dental assistant told me that my overabundance was a good thing and that if I had "dry mouth" , that would be more of a problem. I thought maybe they could extract some saliva from my gums or something, but that wasn't happening. I left the dental office in disappointment.

I'm happy that I did not interfere with nature. My spit moisturizes my mouth in just the way I need it to and it can do the same for you. I've noticed that when I have an urge to suck my guy, my mouth becomes more engorged with spit. It's the weirdest thing, I know, but that shows the level of passion I have for the art of sucking.

You can practice learning how to draw spit towards the front of your mouth. Try grabbing one side of your gum and sucking on the bottom of your lower gum to draw some spit. Like I said, my mouth naturally secretes spit in loads so it's easy for me. Your mouth may be different so if you have difficulties, there are other agents that can help you, which we will discuss in a later chapter.

Once you've mastered the art of drawing spit in your mouth, you now want to share it with your guy's penis. When you are sucking, you

want your mouth to feel like your vagina.
Tight and wet...

Gather a round of saliva and spit on your
guy's penis like a man spitting on the
sidewalk. I know... It seems so unlike a lady
but in this act of passion, all rules are
left at some other person's door. Your door,
with your connection to yourself and your
connection to your mate, is uninhibited at
this point.

Suck on his penis with vivacious spirit and a
smile in your eyes. Rub his penis all over
your face. You are one with it. It shows your
guy that you are in love with it. You should
have a messy but pretty face, and that is an
indication that you are doing your job. If
the penis is super hard and your guy is
moaning, then you are doing your job well.
Some guys like for you to be a little extra
kinky and spit in their faces. That is one of
those fetishes that I mentioned earlier. You
will learn what takes him to the edge but you
have to be open-minded.

As you suck, more saliva will gather,
hopefully in gobs, and you can spit it on the

penis and suck it back in your mouth. Spit it back on his penis, let it run down the sides and lick it back up. Use it for lubrication while massaging the penis and spit a massive amount on the head just to suck it back with that "O" shaped mouth and ever-loving tongue we discussed earlier.

Take some of that saliva and rub it on yourself. Entice your guy by rubbing it on your nipples and then rubbing his penis on them. By this time, your own vagina may be wet so take some of your juices and share them with the head of his penis. If you are so inclined, you could opt to suck on the head afterwards. It's all in your un-inhibitive spirit. The more open-minded you are about your sexual connection with your mate, the more fun and creative you can be with it. It's your call...

## Chapter 11

## The Art of Swallowing

Gag... Gag... Gag... You will hear yourself making that sound of a gag reflex many times until you have mastered the art of swallowing your guy whole. Unless of course, you are a natural born swallower... I had a friend tell me several years ago that her guy loved that she could swallow his penis without gagging. I remember thinking, "Damn, I'm good, but not that good..." Her throat muscles were already attuned to the art of sucking. My friend and her guy are now married...

This chapter is not only about how to swallow a penis without gagging, but also a lesson on how to swallow your guy's cum with delicious delight. You want it to be like eating that pint of your favorite ice cream and swallowing it, while savoring the taste on the edges of your throat. Or that delectable piece of chocolate candy that melts in your mouth while you close your eyes in utter enjoyment.

Every few seconds you are swallowing your own saliva, so it's a natural reaction to swallow when something enters your mouth. I know many girls who are totally against swallowing cum, but they can take a strong shot of tequila to the throat every once in a while. Or down a vodka and tonic all night... If you can take hard liquor to the head, then you should be able to swallow a little cum. Just chase it with a little lime...

Semen or cum, in which we will refer to it, has an indescribable, bitter taste. It is an acquired taste and can change depending on the diet of your mate. Whatever your guy eats will affect the consistency and taste of his cum. By consistency I mean if it can tend to be light or dark in color, watery or milky. So if he is a heavy meat eater, the taste of his cum will be more pronounced. I am a vegan; I know... Kind of hard to believe being that I like to swallow my "meat"; but I can tell when my guy has been eating something he doesn't eat on a regular. I know if I swallow his cum then I have tasted everything he has taken into his body within the last 24 hours. That's some serious love for you...

I get a kick out of sucking my guy's penis until it explodes, preferably in my mouth. The way his penis throbs and engorges is a clear indication that an explosion is about to occur. When this happens, do not tense up. If you do, you will not be able to embrace the liquid that is about to pour into your throat with ease. So welcome it. I want you to think of cum as the flowing, chocolate river as seen in the *Charlie and The Chocolate Factory* movie.

When your guy cums, prepare your throat muscles and let the gush of cum rush through. If you do this with enjoyment, you may not even taste it. Just push it to the back of your throat and swallow. Look up at your guy after swallowing at the satisfaction in his face for pleasing him in the ultimate way. But he will get even more satisfaction knowing that you enjoyed it as much as he did. No matter how sloppy things get, keep it sexy.

If you are a girl that absolutely refuses to swallow your guy's cum then there are alternatives for you. The first alternative is to have your guy cum in your mouth but you opt not to swallow it. You can hold his cum in your mouth and then spit it back onto his penis. You can then take your hands and massage it with the cum. Massage and suck his penis and your guy will be quivering like he just came in from a cold rain. You can also hold his cum in your mouth and let it sexily drip from your mouth as your guy watches in amazement. You're a lady in the streets, so why not be his freak in the bedroom, huh?

Another alternative to swallowing your guy's cum is to have him cum in your face or on a favorite part of your body. I much prefer for my guy to cum in my face. Many guys view this act as being disrespectful but for me, it's a turn on. If you are like me and like his liquid in your face, then let him know just as you feel him becoming engorged. Some guys are more vocal than others and will let you know when they are about to cum, so you just have to know your guy. Speak nasty talk to him. Tell him to cum in your face and more and likely, he will. In those moments, he is so far off in outer space that the closest thing to his penis is where his cum will land.

Look up at him with your mouth open and ready. He is ready to burst in your face and your look of anxiousness will only speed it along. Continue to talk to him. "Cum in my face... Cum in my face please..." This usually will do the trick. When he cums, it may only cover a part of your face or it may swallow your face whole. Whichever is the case, be prepared to get some in your eye, nose, mouth or all of the above. Wipe it off and lick it off your fingers. Whatever you do, please try not to have a look of repulsion on your face. Enjoy it.

If your guy chooses to cum on another part of your body, then embrace it just as well. Make him feel as if he has accomplished a major feat and you are his greatest supporter. If for example he cums on your chest, take your hand and rub it in and maybe even taste a little of it. Remember, keep your sexy.

Happy Head/Jasmine P. Rain

Chapter 12

The Uncircumcised One

Don't be alarmed! There is nothing wrong
with your guy's penis. Yeah, I know it looks
as if things are not altogether attached, but
believe me... It's all good! If there is a
huge bump on the penis, beware! If the head
looks as if it is frothing at the mouth,
steer clear! But if there's just a little
bit of extra skin that's not attached to the
head or it looks like a turtle going in and
out of its shell, there is nothing to worry
about. The explanation... Your guy has not
been circumcised.

The definition of circumcision for guys,
according to dictionary.com© is "the
surgical removal of the foreskin on males."
When a guy exits his mother's womb and
enters the world, the parents have an option
of whether to have the infant's penis
clipped. Although the decision may be easy
for some not to have the circumcision

performed, more so for religious reasons, it may cause the son to have long term emotional and sometimes negative physical effects.

A guy's penis means the world to them. So what a girl, or in some cases another guy, thinks of his penis means ten times more! Does they like the way it looks? Is the size sufficient enough for them? Can I perform to the best of my ability with it? These are some of the common questions that race through the minds of guys when it comes to their penises. So for a guy that has not been afforded the luxury to have full "head" freedom, be more sensitive!

I once dated a guy for 5 ½ years whose penis was not circumcised. I will honestly tell you that the physical fact crossed my mind every time I looked at it. Although I embraced the uncircumcised penis, the lack of growing love that my relationship endured made it more difficult for me to be as accepting as I should have been. He annoyed me. Therefore the sight of his penis was even more annoying. Ultimately, the thought of putting his penis in my mouth was at the end of the totem pole.

However, those times that I did indulge in giving him "head", I learned how to handle the uncircumcised one. By watching how my ex-guy rubbed himself, I took mental note and became a professional at sucking his penis.

In terms of the physical effects I spoke of earlier, there were times when my ex complained that he was having complications with his penis hurting and so after we broke up, he decided to have surgery. Surgery on his penis as an adult! He shared the news with me after the fact and I was ecstatic for him. He even went as far as presenting his showroom shiny, new penis to me on a platter and rubbing it in my face. I was not impressed. I guess he thought it was going to light fire in my ass to come back to him. But what he didn't get was that it wasn't about his penis, but more about our lack of connection. I sincerely needed to move on...

When sucking your guy's uncircumcised penis, pull the extra skin on his shaft downwards and hold it in place with one hand. Begin sucking on it as I have described in previous chapters. Holding the skin in place is important so you won't have to worry about it getting in the way of you sucking the head. Some guys may have more or less extra skin than others. Also, some guys may even want to keep the skin pulled "overhead" while you suck, but it was easier for me to keep it pulled back. Every guy has his preference. Just be mindful of his sensitivities, if any.

Having an uncircumcised penis is not at all a "bad" thing. I don't want to implant that level of thinking into your mind. What I want you to take away from this chapter is that no matter the look, size or shape of your guy's penis, it is a feeling muscle. It's going to always want to explode and it's up to you to learn how to make that happen to keep the excitement in the bedroom. More importantly, it is about keeping your real connection in your relationship with your guy that is going to keep you open and willing to do what it takes to orally please him. Otherwise, I don't care how accepting you are or how good

it looks or tastes at first, it's going to
suddenly begin to look and taste nasty
without that connection in place.

Chapter 13

The Massage and Grip Trip

The art of massage has been around for ages and is a natural healing practice for humans everywhere. When our backs hurt, we look for someone to massage them to make the pain go away. When our heads hurt, we massage them, hoping to relieve whatever pain is going on in the inside. It is nice to have every part of your body massaged because each piece is living and those cells need to be touched. The same applies to a penis. It's almost as if it has a mind of its own. That's possibly the reason guys are always shifting their penises around in their pants or holding onto them for dear life.

When sucking a penis, you could use only your mouth but it is much easier if you grip it with your hands. The sensation for your guy is also more heightened when you grip his penis while sucking. While massaging you want to make sure you remove all sharp jewelry that may interfere with the pleasure of your hand job. I'm a lover of jewelry and will wear rings and bracelets for days, but have learned that during "play with penis time," it's not worth jeopardizing the fun. So I remove my jewelry and if I don't, you bet my guy is in my ear reminding me.

I love to see my guy masturbate. By watching him I learn how he likes to have his penis massaged. All guy's preferences are not the same when it comes to the "jacking of the dick," so it is your duty to learn him. In this way, you will know exactly what to do when it is your time to shine.

Some guys like to be massaged hard and some like it soft, just as in sucking. Or they may like a combination of both. They may like a particular way you "jack it" and I suggest you becoming comfortable with his way. I remember once I had a sex partner and we were newly sexual with each other. I really had not been with that many guys sexually previous to him, but the ones I had been with ironically liked to be handled in the same manner. So naturally, I assumed he would like the same things that the others enjoyed.

During my massage trip, I pulled on my lover's penis in an up and down motion with fervor like I was running a marathon, but vertically. I held on to it as if I was holding a 5-pound dumbbell and in my mind I knew that was going to make him cum to Australia. Boy was I more wrong than a left shoe on the right. He stopped me in the middle of my session and told me to slow it down. To be more gentle... He kindly placed his hands on top of mine and guided my way to the glory of his "nut". He knew exactly what it was going to take to get him there and all I needed to do was to take notes. You can never make assumptions. What you've done in previous relationships may not fare so well in another.

Chapter 14

Peppermint, Ice and Edible Oil

Ok... So now you've had a taste of your guy
and he tastes good. He always tastes good or
maybe not. Either way, you can always add
some spice to his flavor by incorporating
some delicious edibles to the mix. Some guys
may have a little musty flavor in their groin
area, so you may have to nudge them to clean
it up a bit. "Baby, let's take a shower
before we get started. I want us to be fresh
and on point for what's about to go down."
He may oblige and then again he may say,

 "Aww... Baby, you are good just the way you
are. I don't smell you. You're fine." He
clearly does not know the whole time that
it's him you are trying to freshen up.
Depending on the level of your relationship,
you may have to be frank with him. This will
nip things in the bud and get the ball
rolling to some pure and sensual fun.

There are so many things that you can add to
your guys penis to heighten the arousal.

Three of my favorites are peppermint, ice and any naturally flavored edible oil. Not only do they increase the sensation but they can add some added taste to his penis.

Peppermint has been known to have a calming effect. People use peppermints to combat bad breath and it can also be used to heal an aching muscle. Peppermint oil is good for giving a massage in that it cools the body and releases tension. Its use on the penis is helpful in that it gives your guy a tingling but fresh sensation.

A creative way to add peppermint on the penis is to have a piece of the hard candy in mouth. Suck on it just enough where it leaves that "just fresh" taste in your mouth. Place your mouth on your guy's penis with the candy in your mouth. The key is knowing how to maneuver the candy around in your mouth with the penis at the same time. Place your "O-shaped" mouth on the head and suck on it with the peppermint on top. His head will feel a cooling sensation. His urethral glands will begin to rush and it will feel to your guy as if he has to pee or cum. This is a great thing! Continue sucking his penis with the peppermint in your mouth but be careful not to choke. Playing on the playground with candy in your mouth can be a hazard, so use precaution.

You can also take the peppermint out of your mouth and rub it on the head of your guy's penis. After rubbing it on the head lick and suck on it as if you are sucking on a lollipop. It will not only taste good to you but feel ultra-good to your guy. Take the lone candy down to the ball area and rub candy juice all around. Lick and suck. Have fun with it as you watch your guy squirm with excitement.

You can have the same fun on your guy's penis with ice. Yes... I said it! Cold, hard ice... Take a cube of ice and use it just as you did with the peppermint. The ice will be more a little more slippery but I actually like it much better than the candy. You can also use the ice as a form of foreplay. Sexily move it around in your mouth and then kiss your guy with it in your mouth. Rub the ice on your chest and your breasts. Let the

water run down your body. You will be one
sexy chick!

Ice is colder than peppermint of course, but
has the same cooling effects on the penis. It
may have a greater effect and if you don't
tell him, your guy may not even know what
you're using. He'll just know that it feels
good. One time I was sucking on my guy and in
the middle of the session, I excused myself
and made a quick dash to the kitchen. I
opened up the freezer and took a piece of ice
out and placed it in my mouth. I held it
there until I made it back to finish my
business.

When I got back, I continued sucking as if
everything was normal. I instantly heard a
moan that was different from before. My mouth
was now cooler and he could tell something
was not the same. "Ahh... That feels so
good! What's that"? Of course I didn't
reveal the secret until the session was over,
but my guy was more than pleased with my new,
cooling aid.

Edible oils can be used during your "head" session as well. These can be purchased from your local fantasy store or online. They come in all different flavors, so you can have a different flavor for each night! I much prefer all-natural essential oils such as coconut, olive or cocoa butter. They are free of any alcohol-based products and any other products that don't frequent my vocabulary. I also like these oils because they give the penis a very soft feeling and I like the way they give my guy's penis a natural taste but with a hint of nut. They're not too overpowering but they do the job. There are a myriad of essential oils that you can use. It is your preference.

Whatever aid that you choose, make sure that your guy is not allergic to it. Or you for that matter... I would hate for you to have a horrible ending instead of the inevitably fun and explosive one. Oral sex is fun! Using candy, ice and oils only add to the excitement. So use them with proper care.

## Chapter 15

### Driving Him Crazy at 100mph

So your guy is driving and he is looking too sexy for his own good. You're sitting in the passenger seat and feeling like he is looking good enough to taste. The music is adding to the moment and yes... This is the right time to lean over and begin kissing your guy on the neck. Out of nowhere... Tongue him down. Believe me... He will keep his eye on the road but will not know what to expect next.

My all-time favorite place to suck my guy's penis is in THE CAR! Oh... The power it contains and the adrenaline rush is amazing. Plus, I have a fetish for public sex so that adds to the rush. Maybe it's the fact that erotic pleasure is taboo outside the confines of a private place. A car with windows without tint drives my fetish even further, but having tinted windows gives the act a more intimate mood. It really doesn't matter to me. Whatever the scenario, I'm up for the challenge. When I'm sucking my guy in the car, I become somewhat of a savage beast. Something takes over my mind and I get lost in the moment. The sucking action combined with the revving of the engine is a perfect match for me. I don't mind sucking him while the car is at a standstill, but I much prefer when his foot is on the pedal moving us forward into the land of nowhere. I call it that because most of the time my guy loses track of where we're going when my mouth hits his penis. That's the beauty of the control aspect of it. Your guy will possibly be rendered helpless as most times guys curl their toes or shake their feet when their penis is being sucked. So if you're like me and like to live on the wild side, sucking your guy's penis in the car is the way to go.

Once you have kissed on your guy's neck and now stuck your tongue down his throat, touch yourself. Show him that you are horny for him. Get him hot with foreplay action. If it is daylight and the windows are not tinted, be sure that there are not any cars passing by. You don't want to give the cars passing

by you a show or possibly get stopped by the
police for indecent exposure... However, if
it's dark, the sky is almost the limit.

After tantalizing your guy with your
sexiness, lean over and unbuckle his belt and
unzip his pants. Have purpose in your eyes
and keep it sexy. Your eye is on the prize so
you want to be a little aggressive. Look him
in the eyes as you pull his penis out of his
pants because, unless your guy is a fast
"comer", you may not see him for a while.
You will be down deep in the trenches.

Grab his penis and begin moisturizing it with
you saliva. Lick the head and the shaft as
described in the previous chapters. It will
be quite difficult to give the balls some
love since the quarters will already be a
little tight. Your guy's right leg will most
likely be on the gas pedal and although you
want to him to feel the sensations traveling
to his toes, you don't want him to crash
from a malfunction of the brain. I've seen
it almost happen...

Happy Head/Jasmine P. Rain

As your guy is putting the pedal to the metal
and you are high-tailing it on his penis,
lose yourself in a zone. Incorporate the
massage techniques with the twisting motions
and suck that penis like it's your last
suck. Swallow it whole and listen to the
soothing sounds of your guy's moans as he
tries desperately to keep his composure as
other cars ride by. Let him feel on your
breasts or even your kitty cat with one hand
to get him even more excited. When he's
about to cum you will be able to feel his
penis swell and at this point you know the
explosion is drawing near. At this point of
the ride, I'm usually so lost in the
universe that I've blocked everyone and
everything, except for the hard penis in my
mouth, completely out.

As the cum begins to explode in your mouth,
let it pour down your throat. Your guy's leg
will stiffen and his whole body will seem to
want to lock up. Drink up because you want to
wipe the slate clean as to not make a mess on
your guy's pants or the car. Lick every
slither of cum until his penis is squeaky

clean and then lift your head up and look
your guy in the eyes with a smile. He will
love that you were aggressively spontaneous
and that you didn't leave a mess.

Your work is done. Don't be surprised if you
guys are parked somewhere unfamiliar as your
guy probably lost the ability to know where
he was going. It's something to laugh
about... Keep your sexual relationship fun
and a connected spirit to yourself, your mate
and everything else around you and I
guarantee your life will be a happier one.

## Chapter 16

## Shower Reign

For most people, the shower is a private and intimate place. It's where we wash our bodies and gather our most pressing thoughts. Creative juices are born and our fears wash away with the cleansing water down the drain. This is why so many people get the urge to sing in the shower. It's like our own secret paradise where we go to recuperate from all of society's woes. I've come up with my best ideas in the shower. It's not that I wrack my brain thinking there, but it's like as soon as the water hits me, the light bulb shines brighter with every drop.

Every now and then, I like to share my sanctuary with my guy. Taking a shower together is like a taboo ritual that leaves me lusting for the very body standing before me. Watching the water run down his body as he rubs himself in all the right places is like watching soft porn through a Viewfinder. I love showering with my guy because it's

the closest thing to being nude on the beach.
Of course there is no sand, but the sound of
the water in combination with a fine specimen
of a man in front of me has the same effect.
It reminds me of that movie, *The Blue Lagoon*
where the guy and the girl wash all the
unknowns away with a rendezvous on the beach
in the middle of nowhere. It's a reminder
that all the "big" things don't matter.
It's the "little" things that give us the
most satisfaction. Or wait... Maybe it's the
other way around. Ok... It's all
perspective. Sex and water, two things that
soothe my soul, are like cake and ice cream.
They just go hand in hand.

Stand in the shower with your guy. Wash
yourself like normal but add some sexy to it.
He will probably be washing himself as well,
so both of you will be extra squeaky clean.
Massage yourself with your washcloth and
watch your guy as he watches you back. Stand
in front of him with your back turned to him
and let his penis poke you in the back. This
is a clear indication that your guy is ready
for some shower action. If he turns his back
to face the shower head, wash his back with

your sudsy washcloth in one hand and take
your other hand and rub the other parts of
his back. Rub the back of his neck, his ass
and any part of his body that draws your
attention. Begin to kiss his back and take
the hand with the washcloth and rub his penis
with it from the back. Rub his penis with the
washcloth and grip it. "Jack it" and kiss
his back simultaneously. Turn him around to
face you and kiss his lips. Let the water run
down your faces. If you are concerned about
your hair and don't have on a shower cap,
let your guy stand near the end of the
streaming water. I'm personally willing to
mess up my hair and take one for the team...
It's all about the moment. Don't worry
about messing up your hair; what your guy
thinks about your body or your nosy
neighbors. Your focus should be the passion
between you and your guy.

Drop the washcloth. It's done its job for
now. Let your guy suck on your breasts. Feel
the intensity of the water and the heat of
the energy between the two of you.

Kiss him once more then lower your body until your face is staring at his rock hard penis. Begin making love to it with your mouth. Take everything that you learned in all the previous chapters and apply it to this moment. His penis should already be wet enough, so not too much saliva action is needed. Let the penis slide down your throat and suck the head with your juicy lips. Masturbate as you enjoy the freshness of it in your mouth. Look up at him. This is your guy that you enjoy pleasing... The explosion is sure to come, unless you guys have extra-curricular activities on the brain... It is not uncommon for sex to be a follow-up to this act.

You can also try sucking him while he is lying down in the shower; standing up against the shower wall or maybe while you lie down and he sticks it in your mouth. Have fun with it. Your sexual relationship deserves the adventure.

When it comes to oral sex, the possibilities are endless. You just have to be open and comfortable with yourself. The more comfortable you are with yourself and with

your mate, the more you will be open to being
who you really are without fear. Be you! That
connective spirit that you embrace in your
sex life will surely have a positive effect
on every other aspect of your life.
Remember... However you choose to do it...
Keep it sexy! The power of Happy Head is
within you!!

Chapter 17

## The Connection: From the Mouths of Chicks

Writing *Happy Head: The "Spiritual" Guide to Amazing Oral Sex* was an absolute joy for me! In taking the time to share with you guys, I wanted to interview some other chicks besides myself who could share their experiences with giving "head". In this chapter, I have compiled a list of six interviews with chicks that have little to no experience with giving "head" to the professional "head" givers. From the ones who love to give it to those who frown at the thought of it. Everyone has a different perspective on the subject and each level of experience is unique. So sit back and enjoy!

# 36 Year Old Female Accountant

1. Have you ever given "head"? *Yes.*

2. How long have you been giving "head"? *Don't do it often, first time was many, many years ago.*

3. Do you like giving "head"? Why or why not? *It depends. Sometimes yes other times no.*

4. Can you tell me about your first experience? *I don't remember it.*

5. Do you initiate it or does your partner have to ask? *I believe the first time I was asked. But usually I initiate.*

6. Are you passionate about it? *That depends on the moment.*

7. If applicable, what is your favorite thing to do? *N/A*

8. What is your least favorite thing to do? *N/A*

9. Could you live without doing it if your guy was ok with it? *Of course.*

10. Do you have a favorite place or position that you like to perform it? What are they? *No.*

11. Do you gag? Or is it effortless? *Not anymore.*

12. Do you like to swallow or is that off limits? *Off limits*

13. Does his semen or "cum" in your mouth repulse you or are you a self-proclaimed "cum-a-holic"? *Not too thrilled about it.*

14. Do you like your guy shaved or unshaved? *Shaved*

15. What is totally off-limits for you when it comes to oral sex? *#12*

16. If there is something that your guy really wants you to do and you don't want to do it, are you open to compromise? *Yes.*

17. Do you feel a connection with your guy when you perform oral sex? *Sometimes.*

18. Are there any memorable oral sex experiences that come to mind that you can share? *None*

28 Year Old Female Fashion Designer

*1.* Have you ever given "head"? *Yes.*

*2.* How long have you been giving "head"? *Four months*

*3.* Do you like giving "head"? Why or why not? *Yes, only with one person. Because I have to really care/love someone to enjoy it.*

*4.* Can you tell me about your first experience? *My first time was a bit awkward, to say the least. My jaw kept going out on me and I kept somehow biting my partner. I had to learn how to avoid using my teeth on him.*

*5.* Do you initiate it or does your partner have to ask? *Both.*

*6.* Are you passionate about it? *Fuck Yes!!!!!*

*7.* If applicable, what is your favorite thing to do? *This is new for me, only been doing it a few months now and haven't really found a favorite thing yet.*

8. What is your least favorite thing to do? *Swallow.*

9. Could you live without doing it if your guy was ok with it? *Not sure.*

10. Do you have a favorite place or position that you like to perform it? What are they? *In public, in the car or on the patio with light traffic.*

11. Do you gag? Or is it effortless? *Yes, sometimes.*

12. Do you like to swallow or is that off limits? *Haven't swallowed yet.*

13. Does his semen or "cum" in your mouth repulse you or are you a self-proclaimed cum-a-holic? *Doesn't bother me, yet I'm not a "cum-a-holic".*

14. Do you like your guy shaved or unshaved? *Trimmed.*

15. What is totally off-limits for you when it comes to oral sex? *Making huge messes unnecessarily.*

16. If there is something that your guy really wants you to do and you don't want to do it, are you open to compromise? *Yes, I'm open to compromise.*

17. Do you feel a connection with your guy when you perform oral sex? *Yes, it's exciting.*

18. Are there any memorable oral sex experiences that come to mind that you can share? *Yes, sex on the third floor deck. It was complete AWESOMENESS!!!!!!!*
32 Year Old Female Retail Associate

1. Have you ever given "head"? *Yes.*

2. How long have you been giving "head"? *5 years.*

3. Do you like giving "head"? Why or why not? *Yes, I enjoy pleasing my partner and it feels good in my mouth.*

4. Can you tell me about your first experience? *My first experience was very exciting, because we performed the 69.*

5. Do you initiate it or does your partner have to ask? *I initiate mostly.*

6. Are you passionate about it? *Very passionate.*

7. If applicable, what is your favorite thing to do? *I enjoy jacking my partner off, and deep throating with no hands.*

8. What is your least favorite thing to do? *Swallowing his cum.*

9. Could you live without doing it if your guy was ok with it? *No.*

10. Do you have a favorite place or position that you like to perform it? What are they? *69, or when he is driving.*

11. Do you gag? Or is it effortless? *It's effortless.*

12. Do you like to swallow or is that off limits? *I have by accident, but I rather not.*

13. Does his semen or "cum" in your mouth repulse you or are you a self-proclaimed cum-a-holic? *It doesn't repulse me but if I taste it I'll shift and maybe start licking around it or start jacking it.*

14. Do you like your guy shaved or unshaved? *I prefer in between. Not too bald or too hairy.*

15. What is totally off-limits for you when it comes to oral sex? *I'm open and have tried a few things, just don't cum in my mouth! Lol.*

16. If there is something that your guy really wants you to do and you don't want to do it, are you open to compromise? *Yes.*

17. Do you feel a connection with your guy when you perform oral sex? *Absolutely.*

18.       Are there any memorable oral sex experiences that come to mind that you can share? *Yes, I like putting honey on my dude and pretending it's a honey stick, and I lick away!!!*

## Author Info

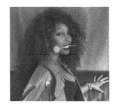

Jasmine P. Rain is the author of *The Social: How Zune Changed My Life and A Light Through The Shade: The Autobiography of a Queen*. She is in the process of writing several more sex books and is currently spreading the word about Happy Head on her Youtube channel, as well as performing her "pornotry".

IG @jasmineprain

 @JasminePRain

Jasmine P. Rain

Youtube: Jasmine P. Rain

Pornhub: JasminePRain

Soundcloud: The Pornotry Ep/Jasmine P. Rain

Blog: www.jasmineprain.wordpress.com

Email: jasmineprain@gmail.com

Happy Head/Jasmine P. Rain

PR/Bulk Orders/Book Club Info: Utopian
Village Publishing

Contact: (404)969-6290

Made in the USA
Columbia, SC
19 October 2022

69749170R00057